Cambridge Elements ☰

Elements in Emergency Neurosurgery
edited by
Nihal Gurusinghe
Lancashire Teaching Hospital NHS Trust
Peter Hutchinson
*University of Cambridge, Society of British Neurological Surgeons
and Royal College of Surgeons of England*
Ioannis Fouyas
Royal College of Surgeons of Edinburgh
Naomi Slator
North Bristol NHS Trust
Ian Kamaly-Asl
Royal Manchester Children's Hospital
Peter Whitfield
University Hospitals Plymouth NHS Trust

RUPTURED SUPRATENTORIAL CEREBRAL ARTERY ANEURYSM WITH LARGE INTRACEREBRAL HAEMATOMA

Samuel Hall
University Hospital Southampton NHS Foundation Trust
Diederik Bulters
University Hospital Southampton NHS Foundation Trust

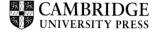

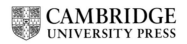

CAMBRIDGE
UNIVERSITY PRESS

Shaftesbury Road, Cambridge CB2 8EA, United Kingdom

One Liberty Plaza, 20th Floor, New York, NY 10006, USA

477 Williamstown Road, Port Melbourne, VIC 3207, Australia

314–321, 3rd Floor, Plot 3, Splendor Forum, Jasola District Centre,
New Delhi – 110025, India

103 Penang Road, #05–06/07, Visioncrest Commercial, Singapore 238467

Cambridge University Press is part of Cambridge University Press & Assessment,
a department of the University of Cambridge.

We share the University's mission to contribute to society through the pursuit of
education, learning and research at the highest international levels of excellence.

www.cambridge.org
Information on this title: www.cambridge.org/9781009517317

DOI: 10.1017/9781009424837

When citing this work, please include a reference to the DOI 10.1017/9781009424837

First published 2024

A catalogue record for this publication is available from the British Library.

ISBN 978-1-009-51731-7 Hardback
ISBN 978-1-009-42480-6 Paperback
ISSN 2755-0656 (online)
ISSN 2755-0648 (print)

Cambridge University Press & Assessment has no responsibility for the persistence
oraccuracy of URLs for external or third-party internet websites referred toin this
publication and does not guarantee that any content on suchwebsites is, or will
remain, accurate or appropriate.

Every effort has been made in preparing this Element to provide accurate and
up-to-date information which is in accord with accepted standards and practice
at the time of publication. Although case histories are drawn from actual cases,
every effort has been made to disguise the identities of the individuals involved.
Nevertheless, the authors, editors and publishers can make no warranties that the
information contained herein is totally free from error, not least because clinical
standards are constantly changing through research and regulation. The authors,
editors and publishers therefore disclaim all liability for direct or consequential
damages resulting from the use of material contained in this Element. Readers
are strongly advised to pay careful attention to information provided by the
manufacturer of any drugs or equipment that they plan to use.

Ruptured Supratentorial Cerebral Artery Aneurysm with Large Intracerebral Haematoma

Elements in Emergency Neurosurgery

DOI: 10.1017/9781009424837
First published online: December 2024

Samuel Hall
University Hospital Southampton NHS Foundation Trust

Diederik Bulters
University Hospital Southampton NHS Foundation Trust

Author for correspondence: Samuel Hall, samuel.hall@doctors.org.uk

Abstract: The ruptured aneurysm with an intracerebral haematoma is a commonly encountered neurosurgical emergency. The options for management of this situation have evolved with the changes in neurovascular surgery training and widespread use of endovascular techniques for aneurysm occlusion. This Element will discuss the differences between subarachnoid haemorrhage with or without an intracerebral haematoma including presentation, imaging and outcomes. The authors present their preferred surgical strategy including practical guidance on how to handle difficult situations such as the intraoperative rupture.

Keywords: aneurysmal subarachnoid haemorrhage, neurovascular surgery, intracerebral haematoma, aneurysm clipping, clot evacuation

ISBNs: 9781009517317 (HB), 9781009424806 (PB), 9781009424837 (OC)
ISSNs: 2755-0656 (online), 2755-0648 (print)

Contents

Typical Case History

A 45 year old woman suffers a sudden onset occipital headache, vomits three times and has associated neck pain and photophobia. Her medical history includes migraines and thus she concludes this episode is a severe migraine. Over the next two hours her left arm becomes heavy and she becomes somnolent. Her husband is worried she has suffered a stroke and calls the emergency services. On arrival the paramedics find her Glasgow Coma Score (GCS) 12/15 (E3V3M6) with a 0/5 left hemiplegia. She is blue lighted to her local hospital where a CT scan demonstrates a right temporal intra-cerebral haematoma (ICH) and subarachnoid haemorrhage (SAH) in the basal cisterns. On returning to resus her GCS drops to 9/15 (E2V2M5) with both pupils reacting normally to light. The ED registrar refers the patient to the on-call neurosurgery registrar located in a neighbouring tertiary hospital.

Epidemiology

The SubArachnoid Haemorrhage International Trialists (SAHIT) group reported 21% of SAH had associated ICH,[1] with a range of 9% to 38% in other series.[2,3,4,5,6] Whilst the middle cerebral artery bifurcation is the classical location it actually represents only 36% of cases.[1] Anterior cerebral artery aneurysms and ICA aneurysms comprise a further 33% and 15% respectively.[1] Internal carotid artery (ICA) aneurysms causing ICH are usually distal, that is, posterior communicating, anterior choroidal or ICA bifurcation. The clinical focus on the middle cerebral artery (MCA) aneurysm is likely because they cause significantly larger haematomas than non-MCA locations (mean: 32ml vs 9ml)[2] and thus are more likely to require haematoma evacuation.

    Aneurysm size is another risk factor for ICH associated with SAH. Medium or large size aneurysms (>12mm) pose a significant risk for ICH compared to small aneurysms.[1,8] Larger aneurysms are also associated with larger haematomas.[9]

History

The history of SAH with ICH can be similar that of SAH without ICH namely thunderclap headache with meningism or sudden loss of consciousness. The distinguishing features with ICH are the presence of focal deficits which are otherwise relatively rare with a pure SAH. Hemiplegia or aphasia from a unilateral fronto-parietal clot would be typical. In unconscious patients a unilateral fixed and dilated pupil may be seen.

Examination

The clinical findings in SAH with ICH are different to those without ICH. SAH with ICH are more likely to be poor World Federation of Neurosurgical Studies (WFNS) grade (21% vs 61%).[1] In the SAHIT series only 13% of patients with SAH and ICH presented GCS 15/15. Another series of 494 patients identified the median GCS of 8/15 for SAH with ICH versus 14/15 for SAH alone.[2] As one would expect, the haematoma volume has a significant influence on GCS with haematomas >50cm^3 having an average GCS 5/15 compared to 10/15 in haematomas <50cm.[3,9]

Many clinical grading systems are used for SAH, including the classic Hunt and Hess and more recent WFNS, and were developed incorporating both SAH with and without ICH. It is notable that WFNS grade 3 are relatively rare, but proportionately are mostly made up of SAH with ICH.

Investigation

All patients will have a CT scan demonstrating SAH with ICH, however we strongly recommend performing a CT angiogram in all cases. It is tempting to prioritise an emergency operation over another trip to the scanner; however, modern CT angiography can be performed quickly and even in extreme circumstances (e.g. a fixed pupil), the risks of delay can be mitigated with mannitol.

The role of the pre-operative CT angiogram in the context of a clot is threefold. Firstly, it confirms the ICH is due to a ruptured aneurysm making the surgeon mindful of its presence. Secondly, aneurysms bleed into the parenchyma where brain is stuck to the dome so they are on the periphery of the haematoma and CT angiogram will define from where haematoma can be safely removed. Thirdly, understanding the vascular anatomy including the aneurysm size, branching vessels and vessels adherent to the dome helps with surgical clipping.

Intra-Sylvian vs Intra-Parenchymal Haematoma

CT angiogram will help discern between a Sylvian fissure versus brain parenchyma haematoma. The primary radiological sign of an intra-Sylvian clot instead of a parenchymal clot is the presence of intra-haematomal contrast enhancing vessels, that is, vessels running through, rather than around, the haematoma.

This distinction is important to help manage surgical expectations. Unlike parenchymal clots, which are one uninterrupted mass, Sylvian clots contain adherent MCA vessels. The clot sticks these vessels and islands of pia and arachnoid together making it much more difficult to suck out. The resultant increased effort to remove the clot frequently results in avulsion of small vessels.

Sylvian fissure clots tend to present with higher GCS and lower volume than MCA parenchymal clots.[6,10] As a result Sylvian clots tend to result in a lesser improvement in GCS at seven days post-surgery.[10] It has been proposed that an aneurysm sac angle inline with the M1 segment is more likely to produce Sylvian haematoma whereas a sharper angle results in parenchymal clot.[6] The latter aneurysms are heavily adherent to pia/parenchyma whereas the former are seen free floating within the Sylvian fissure.

Differential Diagnosis

Any ICH with associated SAH or extending to the pial surface of the Sylvian/interhemispheric fissure/basal cisterns should be considered for underlying aneurysm. Young age and lack of comorbidity also make an aneurysmal cause more likely and warrant CT angiogram before ICH evacuation.

The most common differential diagnosis for the Sylvian clot is a large hypertensive basal ganglia clot extending to the Sylvian fissure. Other differential diagnoses for aneurysmal ICH include vascular lesions such as arterio-venous malformations or cavernomas, or neoplastic lesions. Other causes for superficial lobar ICH such as venous sinus thrombosis, cerebral amyloid or dural fistula are less likely to be mistaken for aneurysmal ICH as they do not extend to the basal cisterns/interhemispheric fissure.

Management

Box 1 Initial instructions to the referrer.

1) Blood pressure should be controlled with a systolic BP <180mmHg to reduce the risk of ongoing bleeding.
2) Nimodipine 60mg PO STAT. Can be started up to 96 hours post-ictus as per BRANT study[7] so patient transfer should not be delayed for this.
3) Osmotherapy. If the GCS is <12 or dropping, or there is a fixed pupil, then give mannitol 20% 0.5–1mk/kg or hypertonic saline 3% 3–5ml/kg.
4) Intubate + ventilate. If the patient has a low GCS then intubate for safe transfer.
5) Transfer the patient directly to the neurosurgery theatre as soon as possible. CT angiogram should be performed en route.

Indications for Surgery

Deciding which haematomas need evacuating will dictate much of your management strategy, and if it doesn't then management will proceed as for a SAH with no ICH with no need for time critical surgery (Figure 1).

The mean haematoma volumes evacuated in other series range from 26–45ml,[2,3,8,10,11] that is, much less than 50ml, with the exception of Stapleton *et al.*[4] whose mean was 100±77ml. It is likely, however, that at clot sizes of this magnitude patients are no longer salvageable. Stapleton *et al.*[4] reported only 36% achieving an outcome of mRS 0-3 and a 33% mortality. Analysis of management decision making in one series found that ICH volume >17ml was the inflection point more likely to favour haematoma evacuation or decompression.[5]

Practically, decisions tend to be based on conscious level rather than clot volume with GCS<12 typically being offered clot evacuation and clipping. Patients in coma (GCS<8) need careful consideration for salvageability and whether to proceed based on a combination of their prior level of function and signs of irreversible injury on CT.

Operative Strategy

We, and the American Stroke Association 2023 guidelines,[12] recommend rapid clot evacuation, which favours craniotomy and concomitant clipping over

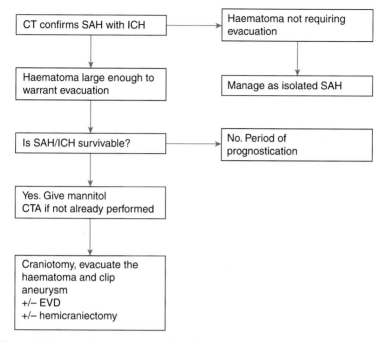

Figure 1 Proposed management plan for ruptured supratentorial aneurysms. Produced by the authors.

endovascular techniques. There is randomised control trial evidence from the 1980s demonstrating significantly lower mortality with clipping and clot evacuation compared to conservative treatment (27% vs 80%).[13] Other evidence from this era showed that clipping with ICH evacuation had a lower mortality than ICH evacuation alone (29% vs 75%).[14]

Surgical Technique

Position – supine with head turned approximately 45 degrees (Figure 2). The head should be extended with the malar eminence uppermost then fixed in a Mayfield clamp leaving as much as possible of the ipsilateral convexity unobstructed to allow for a large scalp flap.

Incision – unlike a simple clipping where we use a curvilinear hairline incision, for clot evacuation we use a larger frontotemporal craniotomy at least the size of the haematoma, often resembling the question mark trauma flap incision. In non-ICH cases we use a subfascial flap; however with an ICH a myocutaneous flap is quicker. If the patient has not yet received mannitol, administer a bolus now. A large craniotomy making maximal use of the scalp flap is then fashioned. The large craniotomy allows the brain to herniate during

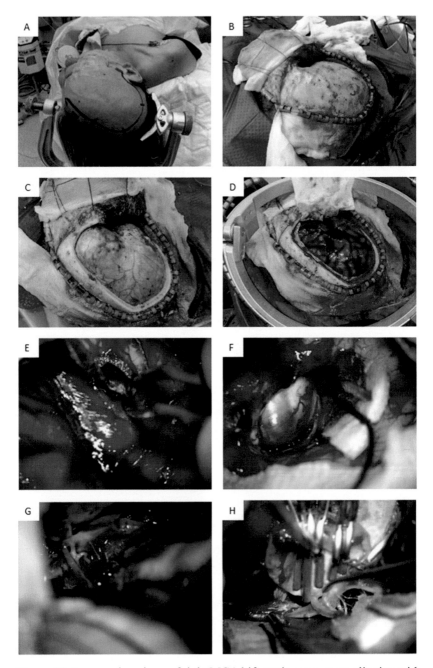

Figure 2 Intraoperative views of right MCA bifurcation aneurysm clipping with ICH evacuation: (A) positioning, (B) myocutaneous flap, (C) craniotomy, (D) durotomy, (E) temporal corticotomy and clot evacuation, (F) aneurysm dome visible through clot cavity, (G) Sylvian exposure of aneurysm neck, (H) stacked clipping of aneurysm. Images taken by the authors.

the procedure, relaxing the brain until clot is evacuated and cerebrospinal fluid (CSF) drained. It can also serve as a decompressive craniectomy if required. The sphenoid ridge is drilled flat down to the meningo-orbital band with a diamond burr to create space to access the basal cisterns.

Dural opening – the brain is liable to herniate quickly so prepare everything for a quick evacuation of the haematoma (e.g. retractor sets and instruments) before dural opening. We recommend using ultrasound before dural opening to visualise the extent of the haematoma and location of the aneurysm within the clot. The dura should be incised in a C shape and reflected against the sphenoid ridge.

Clot evacuation – a corticotomy should be made where the clot is closest to the surface based on a combination of CT, visual staining of the cortical surface and ultrasound. Once into the clot, rather than digging straight into the centre we advocate finding the clot–white matter interface and systematically working around the perimeter from posterior to anterior to remove the clot. This maximises clot removal and ensures you don't lose your landmarks for aneurysm location. The microscope provides invaluable illumination and visualisation of the brain–clot interface. The angles to look fully around the cavity are wide and very dynamic movement of the microscope is needed to minimise brain retraction.

Pearls and pitfalls – whilst in most of neurosurgery a finer sucker makes for a safer and more delicate operation, it is hard to get a clot to go up a fine sucker, leading to use of higher suction pressures and more abrasion on the brain. Instead, use the largest diameter and the lowest suction pressure available. Have a theatre assistant sitting by the suction controls, gently increasing the pressure when clot gets stuck and then immediately dropping it back down. Also make sure you have good control of the thumb control valve on the sucker so you can quickly release suction pressure. A fenestrated tip sucker may also minimise brain trauma. Suggested sucker sizes are: Fr9 for access, Fr12 for haematoma evacuation and Fr6 for dissecting around the aneurysm.

Aneurysm approach – the previously angry brain should now be relaxed. If not, the most obvious reasons are incomplete haematoma evacuation or untreated hydrocephalus. If the brain is slack enough, attempt approaching the optic and carotid cisterns subfrontally to open the arachnoid and release CSF. If insufficient space exists, or it releases little CSF, then insert an EVD (ideally with ultrasound guidance).

We recommend against proceeding with aneurysm clipping before a slack brain is achieved. It is a common misconception that this surgery occurs in a swollen, hostile field. While these patients initially have very high ICP and problematic herniation, removing the blood clot creates a lot of space and in the vast majority will leave a comfortable operative field.

There are two options to approach the aneurysm – either directly through the clot or proximally via the Sylvian fissure (assuming an MCA aneurysm). The direct approach is quicker but has higher risk of aneurysm rupture because the rupture point on the dome will have torn the pia to cause the parenchymal bleeding. It can also be complicated by the pia that is stuck over the aneurysm and its neck and accompanying vessels from this direction. Approaching from inside the cisterns therefore will keep dissection away from the rupture point and provide earlier proximal control. For these reasons we recommend surgeons with less experience approach via a Sylvian fissure split after evacuation of the haematoma and obtain control of the proximal M1. It is important to note that proximal control at the level of the ICA can be falsely reassuring and in patients with well-developed Acom or Pcom arteries in whom the reduction in bleeding from an intraoperative rupture is negligible from a temporary clip on the ICA. Once M1 control is obtained the M2s are exposed before finally dissecting the aneurysm neck in the fissure, with the dome and its rupture point still stuck to the pia.

Aneurysm clipping – clipping can then be undertaken with or without a temporary M1 clip. Our preference is to use one, as it makes the dome softer and more mobile, improving clip placement. Temporary clips can also be used while dissecting the aneurysm neck but are not something we advocate because they cause unnecessary periods of ischaemia and are only for the reassurance of the surgeon. The aim is to have good exposure before dissecting the neck so that any rupture can be easily controlled with either a temporary clip on a well visualised M1 or direct pressure on the rupture point.

After the aneurysm is clipped, indocyanine green (ICG) angiography should be performed to confirm good flow in all vessels and no flow in the dome. All arterial vessels will generally fill at almost the same time and any delay in vessel filling (sometimes just a very pulsatile filling) indicates a significant stenosis. A small jet of ICG into the aneurysm at the clip tips is due to them not meeting completely due to the wall thickness. This can be dealt with either by placing a fenestrated tandem clip across the distal neck, placing an identical second clip above the first or placing a booster clip on the original clip.

Closure – in the vast majority of cases where good clot evacuation and CSF drainage is achieved the brain will be slack allowing straightforward closure. In the event of doubt the case can be closed as a decompressive craniectomy.

Alternative approaches – some surgeons prefer to place a subfrontal retractor as the initial manoeuvre to identify the optic nerve and open the cistern before clot evacuation. This gives the reassurance of obtaining earlier proximal control of the aneurysm. The downside is that herniation of the brain due to the clot (and hydrocephalus and brain swelling) can be an issue and result in retraction injury. Proponents note that while the swollen brain bulges outwards, the sphenoid ridge controls downward herniation of the frontal lobe providing access for a 3/8" retractor. After 2–3 minutes this normally decompresses the brain sufficiently to visualise the ICA (usually with a 1/4" temporal pole retractor) and measure up for a temporary clip in the event of intraoperative haemorrhage. A patty placed at this level will facilitate quick identification of the ICA later in the operation if required. Sometimes the brain relaxes sufficiently to expose M1 (with subpial dissection) and even the aneurysm neck – before going near the haematoma.

Intraoperative Rupture

The intraoperative rupture of an aneurysm is a neurosurgeon's worst nightmare. The conventional teaching of applying a proximal temporary clip or packing both miss many of the nuances that make the difference between a dangerous chaotic situation and an ordered controlled response that allows the operation to recommence unhindered. The following is a guide to help you stay in control.

Don't:

(1) Blindly pack – although with time it will stop the bleeding, if pressure is not applied exactly on the bleeding point, bleeding continues underneath and only stops when ICP is high and the brain is herniating out, making further attempts at aneurysm clipping almost impossible.

(2) Blindly clip – unless you had already obtained good control of the proximal M1 (ideally having left a patty to guide you), avoid the temptation to blindly place a temporary clip. While you may get lucky and slip the clip on the M1, there is a significant risk you put the clip through the neck of the aneurysm or avulse a vessel, which is far worse than the bleeding from the dome you started with.

Remember:

(3) A good gauge sucker is wider than the M1 and can suck faster than it can bleed if placed in the right position.

(4) Direct pressure exactly on the rupture point for five minutes will seal the rupture point and allow your operation to proceed as if the rupture never happened.

Therefore do:

(5) Find the exact rupture point – fight your instinct to rush, instead methodic-
    ally move your sucker in a grid around the area of bleeding to identify
    exactly where the blood is coming from. A two-sucker technique is best
    with the primary sucker in your left hand searching for the bleeding point
    and the second sucker in your right hand (or with your assistant) kept static
    at the most dependent point in the field to stop it filling up. The aim is to see
    part of the dome with a jet of blood coming out, and the jet going directly
    into the sucker with no spill over. Your assistant can then hold their sucker
    in this location giving you a clear operative field in which to work.

If you have already exposed the M1:

(6) Place a temporary clip on a well displayed M1.

If the M1 has not been clearly displayed yet or there is still a lot of aneurysm
dissection to be done that will require a long temporary clip time, instead:

(7) Stick a piece of Surgicel on the rupture point – the aim is to place
    a relatively small piece of Surgicel *exactly* on the rupture point followed
    by a small micropatty before it is washed or sucked away. Once the
    bleeding is stopped you will leave the Surgicel stuck on the dome and
    a smaller piece will get in your way less. The reason for the small patty is to
    ensure that pressure is applied by the sucker directly on the rupture point
    and not slightly adjacent to it (in which case the bleeding will not stop).

(8) Apply pressure – with Surgicel, micropatty and pressure on the rupture
    point the bleeding will initially continue through the patty; however if you
    are applying pressure exactly on the rupture point this bleeding will not be
    apparent as the blood will go directly into the sucker. Hold your sucker in
    this exact position for five minutes. You can lift the pressure off from time
    to time and will sequentially see less and less blood soaking through the
    patty. After five minutes it should be dry on removal of the sucker.

(9) Continue with the operation – at this point the aneurysm dome tends to be
    stronger than you might expect, and the operation can resume as before
    with a focus on obtaining proximal control before dissecting the aneurysm
    neck. The micropatty may be left stuck to the dome, but often will fall off
    leaving the Surgicel with no consequence.

With persistence virtually all ruptures can be controlled in this way, with no risk
of extended temporary clip times. The volume of blood lost in the process is
generally much less than expected and rarely physiologically relevant. If you
cannot control the bleeding in this way, then keep searching for the bleeding

point as in step 5 as your pressure has probably just missed it. This latter technique avoids any temporary clip time and, even when the M1 is visualised, can be preferable if there is still a lot of aneurysm dissection necessary before a definitive clip can be placed on the aneurysm itself.

If you are still working in the clot cavity at this point and want to find the M1 for proximal control, you will need to suck out a small portion of brain deep to the bleeding point to reveal the pia of the more proximal Sylvian fissure and then open this to find the proximal M1. Note that the M1 may be further away from you than you anticipate because the dome tends to be pointing towards you and the aneurysms that rupture at surgery tend to be larger, and hence the M1 can often be hidden quite far behind the dome.

Alternative Strategies

Due to the advent of endovascular aneurysm treatment and consequent reduction in microsurgical clipping experience, a number of alternative strategies have been described, mostly in response to a potential lack of availability of an appropriately experienced surgeon. Alternative approaches include: (1) clot evacuation and delayed aneurysm coiling (or clipping); (2) aneurysm coiling and delayed clot evacuation; (3) decompressive hemicraniectomy with a separate aneurysm procedure.

Clot Evacuation with Subsequent Aneurysm Coiling or Clipping

In the absence of a neurovascular surgeon the next option is clot evacuation followed by endovascular treatment of the aneurysm at the soonest possible time. ICH evacuation is a general neurosurgical procedure which the on-call team should be able to handle. This approach is a tradeoff, which allows emergent treatment of intra-cranial hypertension caused by the haematoma but delays securing the aneurysm until appropriately trained staff are available.

The biggest concern for a non-vascular neurosurgeon is aneurysm rupture during clot evacuation. This is, however, much rarer than most believe and can be controlled as described above. In one series, only 6% out of 398 ruptured aneurysms clipped suffered an intra-procedure rupture.[15] Of these, only two (0.5%) ruptured on opening the dura, three (0.75%) on evacuating a haematoma and four (1%) due to brain retraction with the remainder rupturing during aneurysm dissection. In our own series seven out of 33 clipping + clot evacuations had an intraoperative rupture but only one (3%) occurred on opening the dura and the remainder were during aneurysm manipulation. Thus, the non-vascular neurosurgeon should be comforted that there is only a 2–3% risk of premature aneurysm rupture if they refrain from dissecting the aneurysm.

Following clot evacuation, the aneurysm can be treated in an early planned fashion with either coiling or clipping. While many will go to coiling, it should be remembered that most cases will be MCA aneurysms, a location often associated with anatomy more suited to clipping than coiling.

Clipping at the time of clot evacuation is preferred over a two-stage approach because: (1) it eradicates the risk of rebleeding during the delay until aneurysm treatment, and (2) it carries the risk of one rather than two procedures (e.g. anaesthetic risks and the vascular risks of rupture or vessel injury).

Aneurysm Coiling with Subsequent Clot Evacuation

There are several series in the literature that present coiling of the aneurysm before evacuation of the haematoma, arguing that securing the aneurysm first makes the clot evacuation more straightforward when there is no risk of aneurysm rupture. These series report up to 60%[16] of patients returning to independent living which is promising, although series are highly selective and too small to make any meaningful comparison with alternative strategies.

As might be expected, time to clot evacuation has been shown to be associated with better outcomes in SAH with large ICH.[9] Therefore, given the inherent delay to clot evacuation in a 'secure then evacuate' approach, it must be inferior to a single stage procedure. Given that 'evacuate then secure' should only encounter a 2–3% risk of aneurysm rupture, the benefit of early clot evacuation is greater than that gained by early aneurysm securing and therefore we consider the 'coil then evacuate' approach the third choice option.

Decompressive Craniectomy

Primary decompressive craniectomy is a salvage procedure to reduce the intracranial pressure, temporising the situation without addressing the haematoma or the aneurysm. It can be done in a time-critical manner by anyone with general neurosurgical training without any of the potential risks associated with manipulating the haematoma. The disadvantages are that you commit the patient to multiple further procedures including the endovascular coiling, a cranioplasty and potentially haematoma evacuation. Although it reduces the risk of intraoperative rupture, it still does not completely eradicate it and we feel it is inferior to clot evacuation given that all general neurosurgeons should be able to perform clot evacuation.

Decompressive craniectomy can be used in conjunction with the clipping/clot evacuation if cerebral oedema causes brain herniation through the craniotomy. Adequate haematoma evacuation +/− CSF drainage will usually create enough space to allow replacement of the bone flap in the vast majority of cases.

However, in an occasional case, usually where the clot is localised within Sylvian fissure and good evacuation is more difficult, decompressive craniectomy can be a life-saving adjunct.

Minimally Invasive

Several minimally invasive approaches to managing the aneurysmal haematoma have been proposed. Following coiling of the aneurysm, one option for removing the haematoma is stereotactic aspiration with the Apollo device[17] or aspiration with urokinase irrigation for several days.[18] While these minimally invasive approaches provide promise for deep-seated haematomas, most aneurysmal ICH are large and come close to the surface of the convexity or Sylvian fissure making them amenable to open surgery. Therefore, more research is necessary to be able to judge the role of these procedures in aneurysmal ICH.

Prognosis/Outcomes

It is unclear if the rate of rebleeding in patients with SAH and ICH is the same as SAH alone. Some studies have suggested it is higher in patients with SAH and ICH[5,9,19] and the rate is even higher for clots >50ml.[9] Other studies have not reproduced this finding and report equal rates (<10%) for SAH/ICH and SAH alone.[2]

The presence of an ICH is an independent predictor for worse outcome in SAH.[8] The SAHIT group report unfavourable outcomes (Glasgow Outcome Score 1–3) are nearly double amongst patients with ICH (51% vs 27%).[1] Markers for functional outcome such as rates of return to work (32% vs 13%) and epilepsy (23% vs 7%) are worse in patients with SAH/ICH compared to SAH.[2] The mortality rates in patients with SAH/ICH are approximately 28–35% compared to 15–22% in SAH alone.[1,2,9]

Clot location influences outcome with favourable outcome seen in 48% of temporal clots compared to 36% frontal and 18% Sylvian locations.[20] Sylvian location also has a higher mortality than temporal or frontal.[21]

Clot volume impacts on functional outcome with significantly fewer favourable outcomes in patients with clot volumes >50ml (12% vs 31%)[9] and haematomas >50ml are associated with lower rates of return to work (7% vs 14%).[9] At six months post-haemorrhage (SAH alone, SAH + ICH < 50ml and SAH + ICH > 50ml) relatives felt the patient was exactly the same person as before the haemorrhage in 46%, 21% and 5% respectively.[9]

SAH severity grade is another predictor of poor outcome in patients with SAH and ICH.[19] Even amongst good grade SAH there is still a 21% mortality rate[21] and 50% rate of a poor functional outcome.[4] Other predictors of poor functional outcome are: increasing age, worsening Hunt and Hess score, higher residual clot, external ventricular drain requirement, intra-ventricular haemorrhage and need for craniectomy.[4]

References

1. Wan A, Jaja BN, Schweizer TA, Macdonald RL, on behalf of the SAHIT collaboration. Clinical characteristics and outcome of aneurysmal subarachnoid hemorrhage with intracerebral hematoma. *J Neurosurg*. Dec 2016; 125(6):1344–51. doi:10.3171/2015.10.JNS151036.
2. Gerner ST, Hülsbrink R, Reichl J, et al. Parenchymatous hematoma in patients with atraumatic subarachnoid hemorrhage: characteristics, treatment, and clinical outcomes. *Int J Stroke*. Aug 2021;16(6): 648–59. doi:10.1177/1747493020971878.
3. de los Reyes K, Patel A, Bederson JB, Frontera JA. Management of subarachnoid hemorrhage with intracerebral hematoma: clipping and clot evacuation versus coil embolization followed by clot evacuation. *J Neurointerv Surg*. Mar 2013;5(2):99–103. doi:10.1136/neurintsurg-2011-010204.
4. Stapleton CJ, Walcott BP, Fusco MR, Butler WE, Thomas AJ, Ogilvy CS. Surgical management of ruptured middle cerebral artery aneurysms with large intraparenchymal or sylvian fissure hematomas. *Neurosurgery*. Mar 2015;76(3):258–64; discussion 264. doi:10.1227/NEU.0000000000000596.
5. Darkwah Oppong M, Skowronek V, Pierscianek D, et al. Aneurysmal intracerebral hematoma: risk factors and surgical treatment decisions. *Clin Neurol Neurosurg*. Oct 2018;173:1–7. doi:10.1016/j.clineuro.2018.07.014.
6. Zhang Y, Hu Q, Xue H, et al. Intrasylvian/Intracerebral hematomas associated with ruptured middle cerebral artery aneurysms: a single-center series and literature review. *World Neurosurg*. Feb 2017;98:432–7. doi:10.1016/j.wneu.2016.11.022.
7. Pickard JD, Murray GD, Illingworth R, et al. Effect of oral nimodipine on cerebral infarction and outcome after subarachnoid haemorrhage: British aneurysm nimodipine trial. *BMJ*. Mar 1989;298(6674):636–42. doi:10.1136/bmj.298.6674.636.
8. Jabbarli R, Reinhard M, Roelz R, et al. Intracerebral hematoma due to aneurysm rupture: are there risk factors beyond aneurysm location? *Neurosurgery*. Jun 2016;78(6):813–20. doi:10.1227/NEU.0000000000001136.
9. Güresir E, Beck J, Vatter H, et al. Subarachnoid hemorrhage and intracerebral hematoma: incidence, prognostic factors, and outcome. *Neurosurgery*. Dec 2008;63(6):1088–93; discussion 1093–4. doi:10.1227/01.NEU.0000335170.76722.B9.

10. Lee JG, Moon CT, Chun YI, Roh HG, Choi JW. Comparative results of the patients with intracerebral and intra-Sylvian hematoma in ruptured middle cerebral artery aneurysms. *J Cerebrovasc Endovasc Neurosurg.* Sep 2013;15(3):200–5. doi:10.7461/jcen.2013.15.3.200.

11. Mutoh T, Ishikawa T, Moroi J, Suzuki A, Yasui N. Impact of early surgical evacuation of sylvian hematoma on clinical course and outcome after subarachnoid hemorrhage. *Neurol Med Chir (Tokyo).* 2010;50(3):200–8. doi:10.2176/nmc.50.200.

12. Hoh BL, Ko NU, Amin-Hanjani S, et al. 2023 guideline for the management of patients with aneurysmal subarachnoid hemorrhage: a guideline from the American Heart Association/American Stroke Association. *Stroke.* Jul 2023;54(7):e314–e370. doi:10.1161/STR.0000000000000436.

13. Heiskanen O, Poranen A, Kuurne T, Valtonen S, Kaste M. Acute surgery for intracerebral haematomas caused by rupture of an intracranial arterial aneurysm. A prospective randomized study. *Acta Neurochir (Wien).* 1988;90(3–4):81–3. doi:10.1007/BF01560559.

14. Wheelock B, Weir B, Watts R, et al. Timing of surgery for intracerebral hematomas due to aneurysm rupture. *J Neurosurg.* Apr 1983;58(4):476–81. doi:10.3171/jns.1983.58.4.0476.

15. Houkin K, Kuroda S, Takahashi A, et al. Intra-operative premature rupture of the cerebral aneurysms. Analysis of the causes and management. *Acta Neurochir (Wien).* 1999;141(12):1255–63. doi:10.1007/s007010050428.

16. Tawk RG, Pandey A, Levy E, et al. Coiling of ruptured aneurysms followed by evacuation of hematoma. *World Neurosurg.* Dec 2010;74(6):626–31. doi:10.1016/j.wneu.2010.06.051.

17. Turner RD, Vargas J, Turk AS, Chaudry MI, Spiotta AM. Novel device and technique for minimally invasive intracerebral hematoma evacuation in the same setting of a ruptured intracranial aneurysm: combined treatment in the neurointerventional angiography suite. *Neurosurgery.* Mar 2015;11 Suppl 2:43–50; discussion 50–1. doi:10.1227/NEU.0000000000000650.

18. Kim SH, Kim TG, Kong MH. A less invasive strategy for ruptured cerebral aneurysms with intracerebral hematomas: endovascular coil embolization followed by stereotactic aspiration of hematomas using urokinase. *J Cerebrovasc Endovasc Neurosurg.* Jun 2017;19(2):81–91. doi:10.7461/jcen.2017.19.2.81.

19. Nemoto M, Masuda H, Sakaeyama Y, et al. Clinical characteristics of subarachnoid hemorrhage with an intracerebral hematoma and prognostic factors. *J Stroke Cerebrovasc Dis.* May 2018;27(5):1160–6. doi:10.1016/j.jstrokecerebrovasdis.2017.11.034.

20. Bruder M, Schuss P, Berkefeld J, et al. Subarachnoid hemorrhage and intracerebral hematoma caused by aneurysms of the anterior circulation: influence of hematoma localization on outcome. *Neurosurg Rev.* Oct 2014;37(4):653–9. doi:10.1007/s10143-014-0560-8.

21. Bohnstedt BN, Nguyen HS, Kulwin CG, et al. Outcomes for clip ligation and hematoma evacuation associated with 102 patients with ruptured middle cerebral artery aneurysms. *World Neurosurg.* Sep–Oct 2013;80(3–4):335–41. doi:10.1016/j.wneu.2012.03.008.

Emergency Neurosurgery

Nihal Gurusinghe

Lancashire Teaching Hospital NHS Trust

Professor Nihal Gurusinghe is a Consultant Neurosurgeon at the Lancashire Teaching Hospitals NHS Trust. He is on the Executive Council of the Society of British Neurological Surgeons as the Lead for NICE (National Institute for Health and Care Excellence) guidelines relating to neurosurgical practice. He is also an examiner for the UK and International FRCS examinations in Neurosurgery.

Peter Hutchinson

University of Cambridge, Society of British Neurological Surgeons and Royal College of Surgeons of England

Peter Hutchinson BSc MBBS FFSEM FRCS(SN) PhD FMedSci is Professor of Neurosurgery and Head of the Division of Academic Neurosurgery at the University of Cambridge, and Honorary Consultant Neurosurgeon at Addenbrooke's Hospital. He is Director of Clinical Research at the Royal College of Surgeons of England and Meetings Secretary of the Society of British Neurological Surgeons.

Ioannis Fouyas

Royal College of Surgeons of Edinburgh

Ioannis Fouyas is a Consultant Neurosurgeon in Edinburgh. His clinical interests focus on the treatment of complex cerebrovascular and skull base pathologies. His academic endeavours concentrate in the field of cerebrovascular pathophysiology. His passion is technical surgical training, fulfilled in collaboration with the Royal College of Surgeons of Edinburgh. Finally, he pursues Undergraduate Neuroscience teaching, with a particular focus on functional Neuroanatomy.

Naomi Slator

North Bristol NHS Trust

Naomi Slator FRCS (SN) is a Consultant Spinal Neurosurgeon based at North Bristol NHS Trust. She has a specialist interest in Complex Spine alongside Cranial and Spinal Trauma. She completed her neurosurgical training in Birmingham and a six-month Fellowship in CSF and Trauma (2019). She then went on to complete her Spinal Fellowship in Leeds (2020) before moving to the southwest to take up her consultant post.

Ian Kamaly-Asl

Royal Manchester Children's Hospital

Ian Kamaly-Asl is a full time paediatric neurosurgeon and Honorary Chair at Royal Manchester Children's Hospital. He trained in North Western Deanery with fellowships at Boston Children's Hospital and Sick Kids in Toronto. Ian is a member of council of The Royal College of Surgeons of England and The SBNS where he is lead for mentoring and tackling oppressive behaviours.

Peter Whitfield

University Hospitals Plymouth NHS Trust

Professor Peter Whitfield is a Consultant Neurosurgeon at the South West Neurosurgical Centre, University Hospitals Plymouth NHS Trust. His clinical interests include vascular neurosurgery, neuro-oncology and trauma. He has held many roles in postgraduate neurosurgical education and is President of the Society of British Neurological Surgeons. Peter has published widely, and is passionate about education, training and the promotion of clinical research.

About the Series

Elements in Emergency Neurosurgery is intended for trainees and practitioners in Neurosurgery and Emergency Medicine as well as allied specialties all over the world. Authored by international experts, this series provides core knowledge, common clinical pathways and recommendations on the management of acute conditions of the brain and spine.

Cambridge Elements ☰

Emergency Neurosurgery

Printed in the United States
by Baker & Taylor Publisher Services